How to Boost Your Metabolism Naturally

Metabolic Enhancement Training, Foods and Lifestyle Changes for Faster Metabolism

By

Albert Todor

How to Boost Your Metabolism Naturally

Copyright © 2017

ISBN: 9781520510170

Warning and Disclaimer

Publisher contact

Skinny Bottle Publishing

books@skinnybottle.com

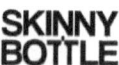

What is metabolic enhancement training

Your body needs energy all the time. This is supplied by the food we eat. The process of metabolism transforms the food energy through the complicated biochemical processes into the forms the body can readily use. This stored energy is released whenever required so that your body can keep functioning in the normal way.

Your body needs a continuous flow of energy for carrying out different functions such as blood circulation, breathing, growing and repairing different types of cells and also maintaining the hormone levels. The number of calories spent on such basic activity is your metabolism. This is also called your basal metabolic rate (BMR).

Factors determining BMR

Your BMR is determined by the factors like the size and composition of your body, your gender, and your age. A person with a larger body or with more muscle mass spends more energy in simple activities like breathing than a person with a smaller body size or lower muscle mass. Men have less body fat and more muscles than women of the same weight and age. So, they burn more calories. With age, the amount of muscle mass is reduced and that of the fat is increased. So, the metabolism slows down with increasing age.

The body also spends energy to eat, digest and absorb the consumed food and to transport and store it. All physical activities like walking, talking, running or performing manual work need energy. Your metabolic rate decides how your body will burn the calories to run your body.

MET goals

Metabolic enhancement training (MET) comprises workout programs, which boost the ability of your body to burn the calories and use the energy produced by them effectively. The goal is to improve the conditioning of your body, grow more muscles and accelerate the metabolism.

The weight of a person is decided by the factors like the genetic make-up, hormonal schemes, and the diet. Your lifestyle, as indicated by sleep, exercise and stress, is also a major factor. When, as a combined impact of these factors, you eat more calories than you burn, you put on weight. You gain weight if you use fewer calories than you consume.

The way is clear; but not easy

So the way to increase your metabolism and to lower your weight is crystal clear. Eat less or consume more by exercising. Or, you can opt for a combination of both. If your purpose of boosting your metabolism is to reduce weight, then keep in mind that the share of the calories burnt during rest, meaning the BMR, is around 70 percent of the total calories you use up every day. This cannot be changed much or quickly or easily. But you can have a good control over the calories burnt through exercise if you have a bit of control over yourself. If you become more active, you will end up using more calories and losing weight, assuming that you maintain your food intake to the earlier level.

So MET includes aerobic exercise like walking, bicycling and swimming for about 30 minutes a day. If you wish to lose more weight, you can increase the total timing of your workouts. You can do these in the stretches of ten minutes, each spread over the entire day. Strength training exercises like weightlifting build the muscle mass and help to overcome the loss of muscle tissues through the aging process.

Change your lifestyle

Lifestyle changes like gardening, walking longer to buy your daily needs, parking the vehicle away from the market so that you walk more, washing clothes and doing household work, can help you to burn more calories by increasing your metabolic rate. But one thing is clear. There is no easy route to weight loss or even for boosting your BMR. You have to work hard to lose every gram of weight and maintain yourself at that level.

The BMR is calculated for men using the following formula:

BMR = 10 x weight (kg) + 6.25 x height (cm) – 5 x age (years) + 5.

The BMR is calculated for women using the following formula:

BMR = 10 x weight (kg) + 6.25 x height (cm) – 5 x age (years) – 161.

This is a rough estimate. But, it is accurate enough to be accepted as the standard calculation of BMR. For the more precise measurement of BMR, you have to go for the carbon dioxide and oxygen analysis after fasting for 12 hours and sleeping for eight hours.

The workouts

People can persuade their body to burn the calories more efficiently by working in the gym. The twice-a-week workout can overcome the slowdown that comes with age to some extent. When you exercise, go for 30-second energy-intensive bursts of activity. These consume extra oxygen and force your body cells to use up more energy. This will also cut down on your exercise time.

The simple job of eating a wee bit less than usual, saying no to your favorite dishes and engaging yourself in some regular but simple exercises often prove to be impossible for a vast number of people. Human beings are supposed to be thinking animals. It should not be difficult for any of them to realize that some things are bad for us and some are good. They must be able to adopt the good things and absorb them as their habits. But not many succeed in achieving this. It's time we all know how easy it all is and how we can manage it if we decide upon it.

Different Exercises/Workouts that can help in Boosting the Metabolic Rate

So, we already discussed that exercise can help you to increase your metabolic rate. But, are you regularly doing the exercises, but still not getting the desired results? In that case, you would obviously be perplexed about how to increase your metabolic rate and reduce your weight faster. Not everyone is born with the body that has a high metabolic rate and a perfect body shape! You might have heard that the metabolic rate becomes slow as the person grows old. However, this sentence may not have made much sense to you. But, it is a fact. Metabolic rate, rather Basal Metabolic Rate (BMR), is the rate at which your body consumes energy at an average temperature and after 12 hours since you ate something. When metabolic rate comes down, your body starts accumulating the food you ate and this makes you obese. And as we all know, obesity and aging go hand in hand. So if you want to stop aging, you do need to keep that BMR reasonably high.

But, are there any ways to keep the BMR high, without using any medications? Of course, there are! And the simplest of these methods is to do some exercises, regularly. However, you must know that there are some exercises that increase the BMR more than the other exercises. Let us have a look at some of the exercises that will help you with the task. But, it is important to learn the difference between the traditional workouts and the modern workouts at first.

Traditional versus Modern (cardio) Workout

Traditional exercises focus on the circulatory system and the way the heart functions. These cardio exercises take some time to achieve the desired heart rate. When the person starts feeling uncomfortable, he or she is asked to step down or continue the same motion for a specific period. You do not have to bother about continuing the exercises in cardio. They do not have to be the low-intensity exercises like the traditional exercises.

Instead, the contemporary BMR exercises are of much higher intensity. They also require the person to exercise the whole body instead of focusing only on the cardiovascular system. Also, there are intervals in such forms of exercises. As a result, these contemporary exercises offer the benefits of traditional aerobic exercises, while also boosting the metabolic rate considerably. These modern exercises also increase the muscular endurance. I am sure; you must be excited to learn about these modern workouts. Let's get into it now:

Dumbbell Dance

You can use a pair of dumbbells to exercise your arms while the thigh of one leg is lifted to a level that it is perpendicular to your body. Alternately, you can try lunge forward with one leg and simultaneously lift both the hands with dumbbells in them above your head. Now, you have to alternate the leg movements to exercise the other leg. You would be exercising many muscles at one go by forcing a higher metabolic activity. Do it in quick succession for almost 30 seconds, and then take a break of 10 seconds. Do it for 5 times as a beginner.

Another dumbbell variant requires you to lie on your back, fold your legs at knees and lift your heels by stretching the toes. Hold the dumbbells in both the hands above your chest. Bring down the arms to the side and let them fold at the elbow while you raise your body simultaneously forming a straight slope from the chest to the knee.

Combination of Exercises

First Exercise

In the first exercise, you can start by standing straight. Then lunge forward and lift an arm above your head. Now jump, yes, jump to stand up straight. Lift the second arm up. This time, lunge forward with the second leg and lift the opposite arm for balancing the jump and repeat the standing position. In the second pair of exercises, you start by standing straight. Then you stand up on your toes, lifting both your arms above your head and joining them at the top. Now you jump and partially squat spreading the arms wide open with the palms facing upward. Jump and go back to the standing position, where you stand on your toes and your hands are raised above your head.

Second Exercise

You can start by standing straight and lifting one arm at a time. After that, you can lunge forward. Lift the second arm pulling down the first arm. Jump to return to the standing position. Lift the other arm and again lunge forward with the other leg. In the second pair of exercises, you begin with partly squatting. Then, spread your arms horizontally, instead of vertically with the palms facing upwards. These exercises should also be completed in rapid succession in a set of 5 or 10. You may take a break of 10 seconds after each set.

Third Exercise

In the third pair of exercises, balance the body on your feet and palms. Then, slowly lift one arm above to form a straight line, effectively balancing the body with the other arm and the two feet. A gentler variation allows you to be seated with your hips stacked. The leg touching the floor is folded and the one above is extended. One of the arms becomes the balancing factor. Now, you can fold the other arm such that the palm of that hand goes behind your head. Then, twist the body to keep the rib cage away from the floor. You may try a variant of this with your balancing arm folded at the elbow. Repeat on both the sides and after 30 seconds; give yourself a break of 10 seconds.

Fourth Exercise

The fourth pair of exercises requires you to balance on your toes and forehands. Now, lift the right leg and take it towards the right hand. Let the right leg go back and repeat the exercise with the left leg and left hand. This exercise also needs to be done continuously for 30 seconds. A break of 10 seconds can be taken after the exercise.

Aerobics

Aerobic exercises include swimming, walking, running and cycling. These exercises are good for improving the metabolism rate. One thing you must keep in mind is that intensity is the factor that determines the extent of improvement in the BMR.

Yoga

Yoga offers many forms of exercises such as Pranayam, Utkatasana, Kapotasana and Ustrasan for improving the metabolism rate. Pranayam and Kapotasana focus primarily on improving the digestion and toning the abdominal muscles. Utkatasana is better known to the west as a chair pose. It includes exercising the abs as well as the muscles in the thighs and other parts of the legs.

Ustrasan, on the other hand, focuses on the lower back muscles apart from the abdominal muscles.

The exercises described above are just a few samples of some contemporary exercises that are good for improving the metabolic rates. You can come up with your own unique form of metabolic enhancement workout with these exercises by practicing a combination of movements and therefore, derive better results when compared to the conventional exercises.

One important tip: Do try all the possible permutations and combinations of these exercises and keep rotating between them rather than practicing the same ones weeks after weeks. This will ensure that your muscles do not get too used to the workouts and thereby consume more amount of energy. It is also a better way to avoid the boredom that comes from doing the same exercise again and again. Rotating between the exercises will maintain the newness in your routine and prevent boredom.

Increase your metabolism with easy yoga and breathing exercises

Losing weight is a tedious job. However, it can be made easier if you have a healthy metabolic system. Giving a boost to the metabolic system is also the best way to speed up the weight loss process. In simple language, metabolism can be explained as the rate of burning the calories by the body. It is an essential factor for improving the strength and endurance of various body organs, muscles, and tissues.

With effective and vigorous exercise such as yoga and breathing exercises, you can improve your metabolism by enabling the larger, stronger muscles to consume more oxygen and burn extra calories.

Yoga and Breathing Exercises to Increase Metabolism

For many decades, yoga was considered as one of the best ways to improve the metabolic health. Metabolism, a biochemical process, plays a vital role in providing energy to the body through the food eaten.

The main organs that regulate your metabolic system include the digestive system, the pancreas, the liver and the kidneys. An improper functioning of these organs can lead to constipation and indigestion. This can further lead to numerous health ailments.

The yoga postures (asanas) and breathing exercises (pranayama) mentioned ahead are quite useful in maintaining and improving the metabolic health.

1. Bhujangasana

Also known as cobra pose, the Bhujangasana works great for increasing the metabolic rate and thus, accelerating the weight loss. It improves the functions of the kidneys, pancreas, liver and the gall bladder.

This yoga exercise is highly beneficial for treating the disorders like indigestion, gastritis, back pain, spinal cord problem and respiratory disorders. It is also the most natural way to cure constipation, acidity, and indigestion.

The Bhujangasana is also beneficial for the patients suffering from arthritis by strengthening the spinal cord.

2. Kapalbhati Pranayama

This is the most popular and a highly recommended breathing workout. It aids weight loss by treating numerous stomach and digestive disorders. Five minutes of pranayama practice every day can provide 100% results for boosting the metabolism and detoxifying the body.

Pranayama is also beneficial for those suffering from heart ailments as it improves the blood circulation and thereby prevents heart attacks. Additionally, it improves the conditions like acidity, constipation, and diabetes.

3. Dhanurasana

This is another yoga posture that helps to boost your metabolism while providing various other health benefits. It works on strengthening the muscles on the stomach, the back and the abdomen. It relieves flatulence and abdominal bloating and improves digestion.

Dhanurasana is also beneficial for arthritis patients as it strengthens the thighs, ankles, groins, chest and the spinal cord. It also improves the functioning of the abdominal organs.

4. Setu Bandhasana

Also referred to as a bridge pose, the Setu Bandhasana increases the metabolism by improving the digestive function. It not only relaxes the body to reduce stress but also provides stretching to the important muscles of the spinal cord, chest and the neck.

This yoga posture is also recommended for the patients with heart ailments as it reduces anxiety and calms the brain while maintaining normal blood pressure level.

5. Crescent Lunge

Commonly known as Anjaneyasana, the crescent lunge pose not only increases the metabolism but also maintains the heart rate. Furthermore, it strengthens the legs while providing a wide stretch to the hips.

6. Spinal Twist

This yoga posture is an ideal choice to increase the metabolism. It works by stimulating the digestive system while also aiding the weight loss.

7. Eagle Pose

This is another effective yoga exercise that improves digestion and increases metabolism. Other benefits of this yoga posture include toning of the inner thighs and strengthening of the lean muscles in the legs.

8. Twisted Chair Pose

The twisted chair pose is yet another effective exercise to increase your metabolism. As a part of this exercise, all the body muscles are twisted for better blood circulation. The basic notion is to improve the digestion and the metabolism through the stimulation of the internal organs.

9. The Camel Pose

Commonly known as Ustrasana, this yoga posture improves the digestion by toning up the abdominal organs.

10. Eka Pada Raja Kapotasana

This is a backward bending pose that stimulates the abdominal organs to improve the digestion and increase the metabolism.

Apart from the above-mentioned yoga postures and breathing exercises, meditation is also an important aspect of yoga. It not only relaxes the mind but also provides energy even when you are tired. Since it is equally important to maintain your mental health for a healthy body and a higher metabolism, make sure to practice meditation for at least 20 minutes every day.

Practicing yoga in the correct manner can bring along a bundle of benefits including improved metabolism, higher flexibility, weight loss, improved skin texture, peace of mind and well-toned muscles. Professional training can further enhance these benefits to an optimal level.

The effective herbs and simple home remedies that can improve your metabolism

Like most other people, I am sure you too would like to get in shape. You can start by improving your metabolism naturally with the help of some simple herbs and home remedies. There are mainly two ways by which you can increase your metabolism. You can do so either by exercising or with the help of a suitable diet.

Metabolism is the process that controls the rate of conversion of calories into energy. You burn the fat calories whilst you do the physical work and even at rest. The rate at which you burn fats at rest is known as the basal metabolic rate or BMR. Improving your BMR will help you to burn more calories even at rest.

Herbs and home remedies to kick start your metabolism

It is always useful to have a handy list of herbs and home remedies as a natural way to improve your metabolism and maintain your overall fitness. These herbs can be used by adding small amounts of them to your daily meals.

Turmeric

This nutritious herb, when taken daily in small quantities, can help boost your metabolism to a great extent. Turmeric contains curcumin that keeps your liver clean and thereby detoxifies your body. This helps to boost your metabolism and ensures that you burn the calories even at rest.

Kelp

This is another nutritious herb that contains iodine, which helps improve the functioning of the pituitary glands. It should be noted that the pituitary gland is the primary gland that regulates the production of hormones that are essential to carry out the different metabolic processes.

Cinnamon

This is a traditional medicinal herb that has been used for centuries to treat several diseases including diabetes. It is an antioxidant that helps to detoxify the body naturally. This herb has been shown to have a negative effect on the belly fat and sugar cravings. It ensures that your body uses up the stored fats by increasing the rate of metabolism.

Ginger

As a member of the Zingiberaceae family along with turmeric and cinnamon, ginger possesses great medicinal properties. It has been shown to augment the metabolic processes in the body. A medical research conducted in Egypt has shown that ginger can improve the metabolism and help a person achieve faster results with his or her weight loss efforts. It also keeps the levels of cholesterol within normal limits.

Yerba Mate

A South American tea, Yerba Mate, is consumed as a beverage. It contains caffeine as well as some other nutrients that can help you to utilize the carbohydrates in your body more effectively. Combined with a balanced diet, Yerba Mate can help reduce the weight by slowing down the process of digestion as a result of which you feel full for a longer duration of time. Along with exercise, this ancient herb can help you improve your metabolism and keep you on track to remain fit and healthy.

Green Tea

The presence of high levels of catechin polyphenols in Green Tea has made it a popular beverage for boosting metabolism. Numerous clinical studies have shown that drinking green tea improves the rate at which the calories are burnt and used up by the body and thereby reduces obesity.

Bitter Orange

When taken alongside with other herbs, bitter orange can boost the metabolism significantly. This herb contains natural substances like Synephrine that are beneficial for improving the body's metabolic processes. It can be found in the Orange peel and is considered as a natural stimulant just like caffeine.

Combining herbs to make simple home remedies

Simple combinations of the above herbs can provide you with the metabolic kick-start that you would love to begin your day with. For example, cinnamon can be substituted for regular tea to make cinnamon tea. Adding a pinch of ginger powder in your green tea can make an interesting and delicious combination that will refresh you and regenerate your body's cells.

Rose petals are said to work like a gentle diuretic that helps your kidneys to release salt along with urine. Tea made with a handful of dry or fresh rose petals can help the body to lose excess water. Even if you do not have a problem of water retention, you should drink this tea as it will make you thirsty and force you to drink more water that will flush and cleanse your body.

Factors that slow down your metabolism

There are some basic factors that can slow down your efforts to improve your metabolism. If these factors are an inherent part of your lifestyle, you have to eliminate them from your daily routine.

• A poor diet that consists of processed foods, fatty snacks and sodas should be avoided. Instead, consider organic and natural foods.

• Lack of sleep can be a big spoiler as a well-rested body enjoys a higher metabolism and burns more calories at rest.

• Stress can have a negative effect on your overall health by causing an overproduction of a hormone called cortisol, which helps to build the belly fat.

• Fad diets that are low in calories can have an adverse effect on your metabolism and hence, should be avoided.

There are no shortcuts to raising your metabolism without the help of regular exercise and proper diet. As diet plays a major role in regulating your metabolism, adding herbs to your daily meals and using the home remedies wisely will help you to improve your metabolism considerably.

Simple Lifestyle Choices that can keep your Metabolic Rate at its Highest

Your metabolism is highly dependent on your body type and it goes on changing throughout your life. It is not that you cannot change your metabolism. A lot of suggestions have been given for losing fat and increasing the metabolic rate. There is no doubt that you can enhance your metabolism by focusing on the workout and exercising. However, there are some simpler methods that can be easily integrated in your day to day lives, which can help to increase your metabolic rate. Here we are listing six such methods that you will not find very difficult in incorporating into your routine life, nor you would have to spare much time for any of them.

Drink more water

Drinking water is the best way to enhance your metabolic rate up by almost 30 percent. Dehydration can cause many health problems. It acts pretty much like stopping the movement of food in your body and causing a traffic jam. However, there is a greater scientific reason for it. If you want to boost your metabolism, drink it cold as your body has to warm up that water and bring it to the normal temperature to suit your body. Effectively, water takes away the heat and the body has to recoup frantically with an intense thermogenic reaction to maintain the body temperature, which is made possible by increasing the metabolism.

Add red pepper in your diet

Red pepper is not the only pepper that can stimulate a thermogenic reaction in your body. There are many other spices that can cause such a reaction. However, red pepper is one of the easiest to procure and sprinkle. Moreover, it blends well with your sandwich, omelet, curries and many other foodstuffs. It would not only add the flavor to your dishes but also boost your metabolism.

Snack many times a day

People who eat several times a day tend to be slimmer than the people who eat three or four meals a day. There is a scientific reasoning behind this. Insulin, which plays an important role in controlling the sugar levels in blood and urine, is produced continuously by the pancreas rather than just 3 or 4 times a day as ordered when you have your meals. While a small increase in the insulin production may occur when people eat some food, this does not compensate for the requirement.

By breaking your meals and snacking every two hours, instead of eating large meals just three or four times a day, you can ensure that a higher amount of insulin produced is utilized by the body. If there is enough sugar sensed in the blood, the body automatically starts losing the food cravings, thereby effectively reducing the hunger and even the need to munch on something. So, six-meals-a-day is the best plan that would burn more amount of fat by increasing your metabolic rate and keeping your insulin level constant.

Sleep well

Caveman had no deadlines to meet, nor a flight to catch. There were fewer late nights too thanks to the lack of electricity. However, now that we have more than the cavemen, we have lost something very precious and that is our sleep. Eight hours sleep does a lot of good to the muscles, which is why the aches and pains of previous evening seem to disappear when you wake up in the morning. Another reason for why your sleep is important is because of a hormone called ghrelin. It is a hunger hormone that the body continues to produce as long as you are awake. This means you would eat more food because of that hormone, the level of which increases when you are deprived of sleep. This in turn, also lowers your metabolism. So, make sure you get a sound sleep of at least 8 hours every day.

Deny yourself some comforts

Clean your home at times in the traditional way instead of using a vacuum cleaner. Try doing water lifting jobs, moving a bucket from one room to another or taking buckets of water outside for your garden. You could also try to lift your groceries as you move around the store. Any small movement can keep your muscles well-exercised and thereby, well-toned without you realizing it. It will keep your metabolism at a higher level even at rest. This is the best metabolic enhancement training that you can have for yourself. Therefore, avoid that grocery cart while you are in the shop the next time. Cardiologists know this secret and that is why you will find them taking the stairs instead of lifts.

Laughing

This would surprise many, but laughter is a great stress-buster. It is a great way to reduce those extra pounds as it increases the metabolic rate. This is because a lot of energy is used up when you laugh and that forces the body to replenish itself by pulling out some of the stored glycogen and breaking it down. Effectively, laughter is an incredible way to burn those calories and bring down your weight by boosting your metabolism. Studies have shown that about 10 to 15 minutes of laughter each day would suffice. That is possible by watching those comedy shows, isn't it?

Slowing down of the metabolic rate is indeed the reason for accumulating fats in the body in the wrong places. But it does not have to be accumulated. The process can be stopped and even reversed by making minor changes in your lifestyle that are neither difficult nor expensive.

The dos and don'ts to follow when undergoing a metabolic enhancement training

Metabolic Enhancement Training might at first seem to be a very complex term, but if understood clearly, it is nothing that tough. What is MET? Well, to be very frank, it refers to a program that makes you do the right exercises, which can help you burn more calories at a much faster pace and also, use the fuel burnt from those calories more efficiently and effectively.

In this chapter, you will come across certain dos and don'ts that should be strictly kept in mind while undergoing Metabolic Enhancement Training.

Let us start with the DO's.

Go on a protein diet, especially during breakfast

Well, do not go for waffles or ice-creams or donuts at a baker's shop. Rather go for a protein-rich diet, which includes eggs, yogurt, etc.

Eating donuts and creams will bring down your metabolism considerably. Do you want this to happen? If not, then say a big NO to such things and go for a healthy and nutritious diet. People who eat protein-rich foods at breakfast end up taking in fewer calories for the rest of the day. So, not just are you burning more calories, but you are also reducing their intake. A wow thing, isn't it?

Stay Hydrated

Do you want your metabolism to run smoothly? Well... Then think of water in your body as oil in the car. Water is highly essential during the Metabolic Enhancement Training. Aim at drinking at least 2 to 3 liters of water a day to achieve the best during your training course. Also, focus on achieving this quantity depending upon the degree of activities you perform daily.

Put on some muscles

I can consider it as one of the most important things that should be kept in mind before starting your training session. Let me tell you the reality. The MET training requires a lot of physical work because it includes multiple forms of high-intensity exercises. Now, for you to be physically active, you must have such a physique that will allow you to do all such exercises. For example, if you are not muscular enough, you will end up feeling tired and lazy all the time and I bet you, you will quit the MET training after a short span. Thus, do those things, which help you to become more and more and more muscular day by day. It is actually a prerequisite for the same.

The above-mentioned Do's are of vital importance if you are serious regarding your Metabolic Enhancement Training. These will really help you to improve your performance to a great extent. Thus, always keep these in mind during your entire course!

Now, let us switch over to the **Not-to-do things**, avoiding which will help you even more to achieve the desired results.

Do not perform the repetitions too quickly

Suppose that your guide has told you to do a certain exercise, which requires the upward movement to be done at a fast speed and the downward movement at a slow speed; make sure you ask what is exactly meant by the fast and slow speed. Ideally, you should perform this task in the time period of 60 seconds assuming the upward movement is done in 2 seconds and the downward in 4 seconds. It will really be of great benefit to you. Do not try to rush into it as you may end up harming yourself.

Don't lift light weights

Make sure you always choose to lift a heavy weight, as this will help you become more strong and tough in a shorter time span and keep your metabolic rate elevated even during the resting phase. Doing lots of exercises with light weight is of no use and does not even promote the muscle growth! Therefore, consider it as your mantra during your MET and use heavy weights only!

Don't lose patience!

During the Metabolic Enhancement Training, one thing that you should never do is to become impatient. If you lose your cool, all your pre-efforts will turn futile and you will face disappointment. Waiting with patience is the key to your success. You will definitely achieve what you have aimed for, but you need to wait.

So, do the above-mentioned don'ts help you in any way? Well, they surely will help you achieve your goals.

Do not take the Metabolic Enhancement Training lightly. Keep in mind what should be done and what should not be and act accordingly. Your actions will govern the results. Give your best and you will get the best!

The health benefits you will achieve with your metabolic enhancement training

The goal of metabolic enhancement training or MET is a combination of fitness and body building. If you are having visions of a muscular body, then a MET program can help you achieve your dreams. For others, MET training can offer benefits that will help them live and sustain a healthier lifestyle. This chapter will provide information on the health benefits you can achieve with your metabolic enhancement training.

MET is beneficial for the following reasons:

- Growth of muscles

- Fitness workouts in the gym

- Healthy central nervous system

- Slows down the effects of aging

However, the main benefit of MET is that it helps to have a healthy body composition that is measured as the ratio of the fat mass to the non-fat mass. Normally, the people with leaner muscles have a higher metabolism. In short, the leaner are your muscles, the faster will you burn the fat.

Weight training to tone the muscles will help you keep your metabolism at a higher level. You may have noticed that people who visit the gym for weight training have varied demographic profiles and mainly belong to the age group of 30 to 50 years. These gym goers are advised to sign up for a MET program so that they can drive maximum benefits from an expert coach. The instructor will include interval training to optimize the benefits of weight training by using the weights as well as repetitions. The older the person is, the greater will be the number of repetitions and lesser will be the weight load used. This expertise of how much weight to use and how many repetitions to opt for can come only from an experienced coach. Here are the benefits you will achieve by undergoing MET under the guidance of an experienced trainer.

MET slows down the aging process

As you grow older, your muscle tissues tend to become lax and wasted. You muscles become slack and lose their toning. Weight training is the recommended way to grow and strengthen your muscle tissues via a regular regimen of weight training and a healthy diet.

Strengthens the heart

MET uses functional hypertrophy training, which is directed toward building the muscles of the heart. The training is adjusted to suit the age, gender and the bodily abilities of the user by the MET trainer.

The American Heart Association has recommended 30 minutes of moderate to intense cardiovascular training to strengthen the heart muscles. However, it is advisable to consult a physician before you start if you have any health issues affecting the heart.

Women's health

Women are affected as they grow older as menopause causes a drop in some hormones placing them at a higher risk for diseases like heart attacks and osteoporosis. MET can help raise the levels of these hormone via increased metabolism thereby reducing the risk of osteoporosis in women. It also lowers their risk of heart attacks by improving the force of contraction of the heart muscle.

Reduces stress-related diseases

Stress increases the risk of high blood pressure. MET can help reduce the effect of mental and physical stress on your health. If you are suffering from stress-related habits like smoking, working out, lifting weights and doing interval training will raise your metabolism and help you cope better with the stresses of life. This will also help you in preventing the withdrawal symptoms that come up during the smoking de-addiction process and help you get rid of the habit.

Improves the coordination of the central nervous system

Research on the effect of intense physical activities on the central nervous system (CNS) has proved that a regular involvement in sports as in repetitive MET weight lifting session can improve the functions of the CNS. The repetitions help build the coordination between different parts of the nervous system and thereby, also improve the various functions of the body all of which are directly controlled by the nervous system.

Weight training increases the heart rate placing pressure on the heart muscles urging them to pump faster to provide for the excess requirement for oxygen. This, in turn, increases the blood flow to different parts of the body including the brain. This helps to reduce the risk of stroke, a life-threatening disorder that can affect the brain and cause paralysis.

The greater the demand put on the muscles during MET; the better is the improvement in the reflex action of the muscle group. Hence, it can be beneficial for those who are interested in improving the reflex action of the specific muscles of the body.

For this type of MET that focuses on improving the functions of the CNS, it is advisable that the repetitions be completed within a short period of time for optimizing the benefit.

MET improves immunity

The absence of disease is not just an indicator of your good health, it also demonstrates how well your body is able to adapt to the environment and resist diseases. Endurance training in the gym, which is central to any MET program, improves metabolism. MET helps improve the functions of the body's central nervous system, the endocrine system and the respiratory system. This way, it helps the body to adapt and respond quickly to any unfriendly external stimulus.

The benefits of MET are not limited to just improving your metabolism. It is a holistic approach to building the muscles and for achieving better health and fitness. It encompasses weight lifting as in functional hypertrophy training and also a suitable diet. MET is a preventive measure that can balance the falling anabolism and the rising catabolism that occur with aging. Further, a higher metabolism assures leaner muscles and greater immunity from diseases like cancer, high blood pressure, heart disease and diabetes. It helps reduce stress and can enable you to enjoy a healthier lifestyle even as you age.

Conclusion

In order to maximize the benefits of your metabolic enhancement training or MET, you need to have a plan that will include proper diet, exercise and lifestyle. This will help you focus your efforts and adjust to the MET plan successfully.

In the introduction to his book "Cracking the metabolic code", author James B. LaValle very astutely points out that most chronic diseases cannot be treated only with a pill. Diseases like high blood pressure, creeping cholesterol, cancer and diabetes are a result of a human being's sum total of life's habits and lifestyle that leads to a gradual slowing down of the body's metabolism.

Metabolism is a chemical process consisting of two parts. One part is anabolism or the building of the muscle tissue. The other part known as catabolism involves conversion of the food you eat into the calories that are required by the body to carry out its activities. The sum of these two processes helps you build strength and stamina on one hand and slows down the aging process by increasing your immunity to many diseases on the other.

Fitness is the cornerstone of a good MET plan. Most people have different types of metabolism. This simply means that some people burn calories faster than others. The slow burners have to make more efforts to burn the calories they eat to prevent putting on weight.

Here are the summary of various aspects of a MET plan that can work toward improving your health and lifestyle.

Exercise

When you move, you burn calories. If you choose to burn the calories at a higher rate with the intent to lose weight, you will need to do serious cardio training, which will increase your heart rate and spike your metabolism.

There are many different cardio training regimens with each having its own intensity that can boost the metabolism in varying degrees and affect your body in varying ways. Some will strengthen the heart muscles, some will burn the calories faster and yet, others will improve the way the body burns fat. These factor the metabolic training into many different zones with each having its own specific purpose and goals.

Aerobic training

Thirty minutes of brisk walking can burn the same number of calories that you do when spending much less time on the treadmill. Cycling and jogging are other types of exercises that can burn as much as 360 calories when done at a moderate pace uphill for thirty minutes.

Weight lifting as a form of cardio training

In order to retain the benefits of aerobic exercises, one has to spend some time doing weight lifting to build and strengthen the muscles. This type of training may not burn as many calories as aerobic training or help you lose weight rapidly. But if you have lost weight and would like to continue having a higher metabolism, building the muscles will help you in the long run. On an average, putting on five pounds of muscles can help you burn up to 30 calories more daily.

Without muscles, your metabolism will tend to fall and you will end up adding back the weight you have lost.

Diet & Nutrition

There are two parts to a good nutrition plan and it comprises of what and when you eat. Besides, you should eat only as much as you can digest. If your daily intake is 3000 calories and you can eat it all at once without heartburn, you can do so. But, if you plan to lose 3500 calories a week, you will need to eat 500 fewer calories every day. This is some of the math you will need to do to track your progress.

Nutrition is required to execute a MET plan successfully. You will need to eat wholesome foods and avoid the processed foods and sweetened beverages completely. A large part of the nutrition has to come from the food triangle with the correct balance of proteins, dairy, staples and vegetables. Eating from all the food groups is a necessity for good health and building muscle.

If you starve and exercise, you may end up losing muscle mass. Further, eating a high protein diet has not been recommended by the American Heart Association as it is considered to be unbalanced. You should consult a doctor when planning to go for a special diet.

Lifestyle

Leading an active life is the best way to elevate your metabolic rate. Walking and doing work around the house will help you burn the calories without even having to visit a gym. Bursts of vigorous activity done continuously for 30 minutes daily will improve your metabolism considerably.

As you age, nature in its own ways can deteriorate your metabolism. After the age of 60, muscles tend to waste at the rate of 3 to 6 percent per annum. It is a good idea to weight train regularly to build the muscles to counter the wasting of muscles.

A lifestyle that is naturally bound to your daily activities, including adequate sleep, eating nutritious foods and exercising regularly will help you keep up with your MET plan.

You will be able to optimize the benefits from a good MET plan when you gradually adjust your lifestyle to reflect the elements of the plan. This means that you begin to eat healthier, exercise more often and work toward living a life that is stress-free. The best way to begin your way into a new, healthier life is to start today. So, do not wait further. Take the first step in the right direction and boost your metabolism to stay healthier and longer.

Wish you good luck!

Win a free

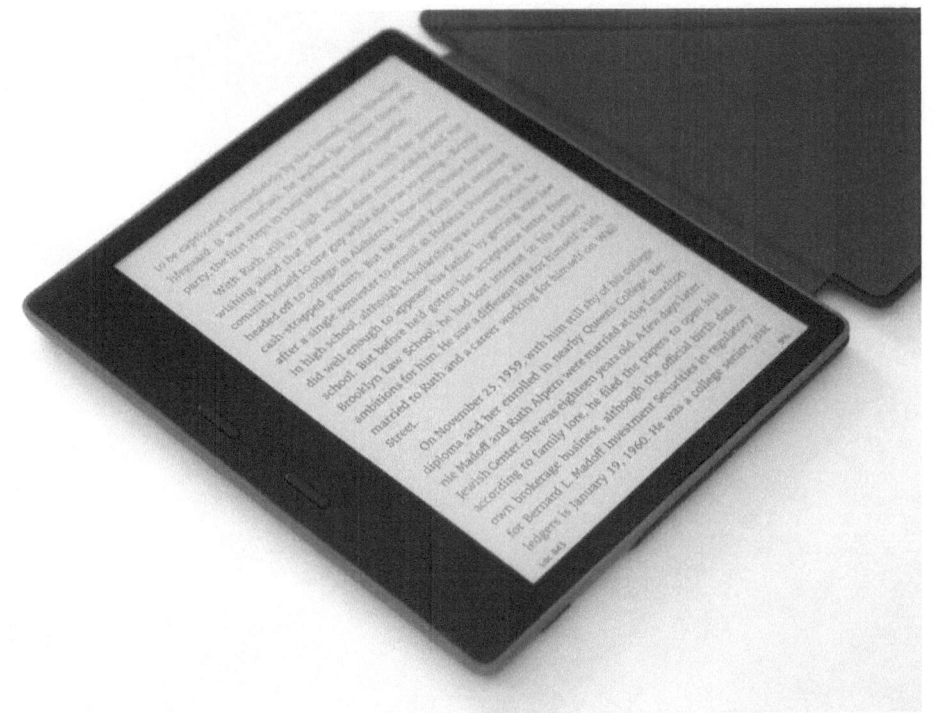

kindle
OASIS

Let us know what you thought of this book to enter the sweepstake at:

http://booksfor.review/boostmetabolism

www.ingramcontent.com/pod-product-compliance
Lightning Source LLC
Chambersburg PA
CBHW030546290526
45786CB00004B/1892